Y0-BDH-759

Manpo-kei™

The Art and Science of
Step Counting

*How to be
naturally active and*

*lose
weight!*

Catrine Tudor-Locke, Ph.D

Dedication

This one is for Gehr-Bear.

© Copyright 2003 Manpo-Kei, Inc. All rights reserved.

Manpo-Kei is a trade mark of Manpo-Kei Inc.

No part of this publication may be reproduced, stored in a retrieval system, or transmitted, in any form or by any means, electronic, mechanical, photocopying, recording, or otherwise, without the written prior permission of the author.

National Library of Canada Cataloguing in Publication Data

Tudor-Locke, Catrine, 1963-
        Manpo-kei : the art and science of step counting / Catrine Tudor-Locke.

Includes index.
ISBN 1-55395-481-5

        1. Fitness walking. 2. Pedometers. I. Title.

RA781.65.T82 2002   613.7'176   C2003-900141-5

TRAFFORD

This book was published *on-demand* in cooperation with Trafford Publishing. On-demand publishing is a unique process and service of making a book available for retail sale to the public taking advantage of on-demand manufacturing and Internet marketing. **On-demand publishing** includes promotions, retail sales, manufacturing, order fulfilment, accounting and collecting royalties on behalf of the author.

Suite 6E, 2333 Government St., Victoria, B.C. V8T 4P4, CANADA
Phone   250-383-6864   Toll-free 1-888-232-4444 (CA & US)
Fax   250-383-6804   E-mail sales@trafford.com
Web site   www.trafford.com
TRAFFORD PUBLISHING IS A DIVISION OF TRAFFORD HOLDINGS LTD.
Trafford Catalogue #02-1196   www.trafford.com/robots/02-1196.html

10   9   8   7   6   5   4   3   2

Acknowledgements

The trouble with writing an acknowledgements section is that inevitably someone is disappointed that they were not singled out in some manner. My fear is made worse due to the fact that I am, indeed, indebted to a multitude of people in numerous regions as I have traveled and grown intellectually and emotionally. Merely listing a roster of names would fill more than a few pages. Regardless of my fear however, there are a few people and organizations I do want to mention; their impact on me and the ideas in this book have been tremendous. First, I would like to acknowledge Dr. Anita Myers of the Department of Health Studies and Gerontology at the University of Waterloo, my PhD mentor and friend, for never being satisfied with mediocrity and for feeding me many chicken sandwiches over the course of my training. I would also like to acknowledge all the faculty, staff, and participants at the Canadian Centre for Activity and Aging and the University of Western Ontario for all their abundant support, both instrumental and emotional. I must also acknowledge the contributions of the practitioners, staff, and participants at the Lawson Diabetes Center; many of these folks were among the first who obliged me by agreeing to wear a pedometer and telling me of their experiences. I also wish to thank Dr. Barbara Ainsworth of the Prevention Research Center at the University of South Carolina for expanding my experiences vastly and therefore my understanding. Finally, I would like to thank my dear friend Noreen Stadey for challenging me to be a better writer and Derek Sarty for agreeing to design this book just because it interested him.

Forward by Dr. Yoshiro Hatano

Dr. Hatano has studied the health benefits of measured walking programs for 25 years, and has been instrumental in the development of today's accurate, inexpensive pedometers.

The 1964 Tokyo Olympics focused attention on fitness and heightened awareness that regular exercise could help prevent hypertension, stroke, diabetes and obesity. Around this same time, modern pedometers arrived on the scene. The convergence of these two events sparked a passion for exercise, walking and pedometer use that has remained a part of Japanese life ever since.

Manpo-kei means 10,000 steps meter and became a popular slogan for Japanese walking clubs. The idea was so successful that today Manpo-kei is practiced throughout Japan and over 7,000,000 pedometers are sold yearly. You'll find at least two of these instruments in most Japanese households.

Now Manpo-kei has come to North America and a number of leading exercise researchers, and health and fitness practitioners are presently engaged in active pedometer-based research and promotional activities. It is my great pleasure to congratulate Dr. Catrine Tudor-Locke on this very accessible, easy-to-use introduction to Manpo-kei. Her abundant gifts as a researcher and talent as a teacher will motivate interested readers to increased physical activity, help them lose weight and enhance their lives for years to come - one step at a time.

Dr. Yoshiro Hatano, Professor
Kyushu University of Health and Welfare, Japan

Manpo-kei Contents

As overheard at a coffee shop not so very long ago—

Susan : (to the service staff): Make that milk instead of cream, please. *(to her companion):* I'm trying to cut down a bit. I'm sick about my weight.

Judith: You're not the only one. I need to do something too. Have you heard about Manpo-kei?

Susan: Manpo-who?

Judith: Manpo-kei. It's a Japanese word. It's about using a pedometer to keep track of your daily activity.

Susan: A pedometer—you mean one of those gadgets you wear at your waist that measures how far you walk? I thought they weren't supposed to be very accurate.

Judith: Yes, a pedometer—but it doesn't really measure how far you walk—it counts how many steps you take in a day— and the modern ones are actually very accurate. Manpo-kei is a pedometer-based program that is all about setting goals for steps/day and steadily working towards them. It sounds like a lot of fun.

Susan: It sounds like exercise.

Judith: No, it's not about exercise—well, it's not necessarily about exercise. You set your goals and figure out your own strategies for getting there. You know, walking more at work, errands, chores around the house—stuff like that. The pedometer just helps you keep track of it all. It's all about choice. Everyone chooses different goals and different strategies, whatever works best for them.

Susan: Still sounds a bit silly. What's the point?

Judith: The point is, we're all couch potatoes, more than ever. We drive everywhere, take escalators—that stuff is nothing new. But all that inactivity every day, day after day, adds up. And we're getting fatter! Practicing Manpo-kei just allows you to get feedback on your daily activity choices.

Susan: Hmm. I have noticed that I've slowly gained weight over the years. I know I'm busy—but I wonder how many steps I take in a day. Tell me more.

Judith: That's about all I know right now. But there is a book out now that explains how it works. I plan to read it—you should too.

The ⊙besity Epidemic & Why It Is Happening

We're in the midst of a worldwide obesity epidemic (1). Research tells us that here in the U.S., 55% of the adult population is either overweight or obese.

But you don't have to take researchers' word for it; go to any place where a lot of people gather (like a mall or movie theatre) and you'll see for yourself that there seems to be a high proportion of overweight people. If more body fat just meant buying larger clothing sizes, it wouldn't be such a problem. But overweight and obesity are well known to be associated with premature death, and many chronic diseases including heart and vascular diseases, diabetes, postmenopausal breast cancer, and osteoarthritis. Ill health is only part of the price we pay. The economic costs totaled 70 billion dollars in 1995 in the U.S (2). And I won't even begin to go into the social and psychological costs of overweight and obesity.

So, why are we in the middle of an obesity epidemic when we live in a society that values being thin? What has changed in the past few decades that has had such a negative impact on the health of so many people? There are likely many contributing social and environmental factors, but it all comes down to a positive energy imbalance, that is, energy-in exceeding energy-out. A positive energy imbalance leads to weight gain over time. Basically, if you take in more (eat more) than you expend, you gain weight. Or to put the emphasis somewhat differently, if you expend less than you take in, you gain weight. So the recipe for an obesity epidemic would seem to be eating too much (and/or making poor choices including high fat foods) and not exercising. Oddly, however, researchers are telling us that we eat less than our predecessors, that consumption of high fat foods has decreased over time and that participation in leisure-time physical activity (sports and exercise) has remained relatively stable (3). Yet we continue to become fatter. Such a confusing situation has been referred to as the "American Paradox (4)."

So what is really going on? I suspect that this obesity epidemic is due to eating too much and/or making inappropriate choices relative to a diminishing energy-out side of the equation. This latter factor bears closer scrutiny. Although participation in intentional leisure-time physical activities has remained stable, incidental activities, or opportunities to be naturally active on a daily basis, have dwindled over the last four decades. What do I mean by naturally active? Being naturally active goes beyond exercising for its own sake—it includes energy expended throughout the day in incidental work activities, chores, childcare, errands, commuting, etc. Think of it as the minimal level of background activity necessary for daily living. For example, going for a walk for its own sake would be classified as exercise, or an intentional activity—but walking as a means of short distance transportation is an incidental activity—that is, being naturally active. Both examples of walking expend energy and are related to a host of health benefits—only the purpose for the walking differs: incidental transportation vs. intentional exercise. The need to be naturally active has eroded without much notice until now. I believe that walking (regardless of form or purpose) has been especially susceptible to the ravages of modernization. I also believe that the loss of background activity necessary for daily living (or natural activity) is a major contributor to the obesity epidemic—making eating even modest amounts and infrequent high fat delicacies too much to handle without creeping weight gain.

Sedentarism is a feature of modern life. Sedentarism is a lifestyle marked by much physical inactivity and relatively little physical activity. Physical inactivity has been defined by researchers as "a state in which bodily movement is minimal (15)." Behaviors considered to be physically inactive are extremely common and include: sleeping, eating, standing still (e.g., waiting in line), sitting, watching television, reading, working on a computer, talking on a phone, and passive commuting (e.g., riding in a car) (5,6). The U.S. Surgeon General (3) has stipulated that physical inactivity is a major health risk factor. Research estimates that between 54% and 60% of the adult population is not "sufficiently active" to achieve health benefits and 25% may be "completely sedentary" or "not active at all (3,7)."

On a more positive note, the benefits of increased physical activity are well documented, and include weight loss and maintenance, reduced risk of chronic disease, and improved quality of life. In short, physical activity is good for you.[1] But most people who are practiced in the art of sedentary daily living find that adopting and maintaining a structured and regimented exercise program is exceedingly difficult to do. How many times have you started an exercise program? And don't feel guilty about your answer—you're not alone. One often-cited finding is that about 50% of aerobics class joiners drop out in the first 3-6 months, most in the first 12 weeks (10). In fact, it is so difficult to keep up with an exercise routine that a whole branch of research has sprung up to study exercise adoption and adherence behavior!

[1] *A special note for those who smoke...*

I won't quibble about this: if you smoke, the best thing you can do for your health is quit. In saying that, I also recognize that quitting smoking is one of the most difficult behavior changes you can make. Since the health benefits are so overwhelming, I whole-heartedly encourage you to try, and keep trying, to quit.

In the meanwhile, I hope you'll be encouraged to know that research evidence suggests that for those who smoke, moderate and high levels of physical fitness provide some protection from death due to cardiovascular disease (8). On the flip side, a low level of physical fitness has been described as a precursor of mortality in smokers. So, if you smoke, you are even more in need of a practical and effective activity intervention (9). If you don't necessarily savor the idea of structured exercise, you are reading the right book!

If you think that signing up for an aerobics class or committing to training for a marathon are the only ways to reap the benefits of a physically active lifestyle, think again. Walking, regardless of form or purpose, qualifies as an appropriate physical activity. In 1996 the U.S. Surgeon General endorsed a public health recommendation to accumulate 30 minutes or more of moderate intensity activity (like brisk walking) on most, if not all, days of the week (3,11). Taken literally, the Surgeon General's recommendation implies we only need to track our time in such activity using a wristwatch and add up all the separate bouts throughout the day. This is impractical. While timepieces may be useful for tracking continuous bouts of intentional exercise (e.g., running for 40 minutes) it is ridiculous to consider timing and adding up all the incidental walking related to errands, chores, childcare, active commuting, etc. The mental image makes me giggle! What I propose is a more practical and palatable approach to naturally increasing and systematically tracking daily physical activity— especially walking or what research-types call ambulatory activity. The approach I recommend is amenable to individual preferences, abilities, and schedules. It does not require a great deal of planning or expense. Importantly, it does not dismiss the concept of intentional exercise, just builds it in as one of the many optional strategies for increasing daily physical activity. I call this approach Manpo-kei: the art and science of step counting. But before I give it all away, let me try to convince you further of the merits of such a simple approach to reclaiming your natural activity.

The Evolution of Physical Inactivity

In the beginning, we were naturally physically active. Although games and sport were recognized as part of daily life, exercise as a purposeful activity of its own was an alien concept.

Hunting, gathering, farming, building shelter, traveling, and preparing food were all demanding physical activities. Throughout the day we had a need to move, to walk, to bend, to reach, to jump, to push, to pull, to lift. We needed to bang laundry on rocks, forage for firewood, dig up root vegetables, and migrate seasonally pulling everything with us. Life wasn't easy—and getting enough exercise was not an issue.

So we began to make life easy by inventing and collecting gadgets. Labor-saving or energy-sparing gadgets. Throughout the ages, we've displayed our ingenuity beginning with the invention of the wheel in the stone age, gaining momentum with the invention of the conveyor belt in the industrial age, and reaching a pinnacle now with the computer chip of the digital age. Today, all we need to do is double-click, punch buttons on a phone, a bank machine keypad or a remote control, and know how to drive a car with an automatic transmission. We live in a time and society characterized by little necessity to expend energy for survival on a daily basis. Opportunities for natural physical activity are on the endangered list. The motor vehicle, whatever we choose to drive, reigns supreme. People-movers of all kinds—cars, courtesy shuttles, escalators, take us where we want to go, and doors open automatically when we get there! And with the growing trends for home-based offices, computer shopping, and home entertainment systems, we soon won't need to walk anywhere at all. Now life is easy—but getting enough exercise is definitely an issue!

Enlightened researchers and health professionals have recognized the detrimental health effects of this trend towards sedentarism and have recommended various forms of structured exercise as a compensatory strategy. However, given how pervasive inactivity is nowadays, exercise can be too feeble an attempt to reconcile the daily deficit of energy-out. For example, engaging in structured exercise like walking on a treadmill a couple times a week just can't possibly compete with the magnitude of inactivity inherent in modern life. I suspect that no piece of exercise equipment—no matter what the infomercial says—can save you (unless you stay on it a very, very, long time). We've made life so easy that it is also easy to become obese, easy to develop cardiovascular disease and diabetes, and easy to die before our time.

Let me illustrate by describing a typical day in the life of one imaginary individual (realize that I'm exaggerating a bit to drive home my points, but hopefully you will still find this case study recognizable). Susan begins the morning by hitting the snooze button to extend her repose but eventually gives in and gets up. While her husband lets the dog out into the back-yard, Susan steps on the weight scale. She scowls and resolves to do something about it. She enjoys a sensible breakfast then rallies the troops into the standard-issue mini-van after kissing her husband goodbye and sending him off in another direction for the day. Susan drives the children six blocks to school (gets caught in the daily traffic-jam of anxious parents surrounding the school), then makes a series of quick stops at the drive-through bank machine, the drive-through cleaners, the drive-through video store drop-box, and her favorite drive-through coffee shop. At the coffee shop the traffic line-up is long and she momentarily considers getting out of the van and going inside to get her coffee, but she just can't be bothered. She enters the ritual of gridlock traffic steadily edging itself towards the city center. She's mildly aware that most of the vehicles carry only a driver and no passengers. Susan parks in her assigned spot, takes the parking shuttle to her office building, takes the elevator to the second floor and settles into her cubicle with the ergonomically-correct office chair and computer keyboard. She commands the world from this keyboard and monitor. In fact, Susan communicates with others in the same office via e-mail rather than walking down the hall for a face-to-face meeting. The only breaks she takes for the morning are a quick trip to the coffee machine and another to the little girls room. She sometimes eats lunch downstairs in the food court but today she orders in (again, choosing sensibly) so she can keep focused on her work. By the end of her workday Susan is mentally exhausted having dealt with phones, e-mail messages, faxes, and deadlines. She is relieved that her husband is in charge of picking the kids up from their computer club after school. This allows her time to drop into her favorite fitness club. She generally aims to hit the club three days a week, but more often than not it is two or fewer days a week. Susan does some stretching exercises while she waits 15 minutes for her name to come up on the treadmill sign-in sheet. Then she walks briskly for 20 minutes (the club's limit during peak times) while catching the last part of "Oprah" on a suspended television. Filled with a sense of having accomplished her exercise goal, she gets back in the mini-van and joins the slow-moving parade back home. She makes a quick stop at the video store for the evening's entertainment and gets mildly annoyed with having to park farther away from the door than she might like. On the way home, she decides to wash the mini-van at the new drive-through car wash. Susan arrives home to find the kids playing video games and her husband just finishing the lawn with his riding mower. Inside, she wonders how anyone could have lived without microwaves, dishwashers, and washers and dryers. And she promises herself once again that she will someday have a maid to do all the housework. The family devours supper (sensible, of course) in front of the TV, watching the video-pick. There is momentary confusion about which of the many remote controls are required to operate the VCR. After the flick, her husband lets the dog out into the backyard while the kids get ready for bed. Susan falls asleep on the couch watching the news with her husband. The routine plays out much the same way, week after week. A month later Susan steps on the weight scale, scowls and resolves to do something about it. She notices that her husband and kids are getting a little more rotund too.

So what's going on here? Our heroine is eating right and exercising. And yet the fat won't go away—in fact she seems to be gaining weight! Susan's problem is shared with many people in today's society. The problem is that our lifestyle has evolved to a level where opportunities for natural physical activity are as rare as hen's teeth. And sporadic attempts at structured exercise seem futile in the face of such sloth. We suffer the consequences with creeping obesity—the imperceptibly slow accumulation of unwanted body fat that seems amazingly resistant to our most concerted attempts to block or shed it.

All is not lost, however. It's time to take back our naturally active lives. I'm not suggesting we go back to banging our laundry on rocks. Really, I'm quite delighted to be living in this day and age and there is no way I'm giving up my washer and dryer. But given the situation, we need to consider becoming more aware of opportunities for natural activity that exist in our lives, tracking our daily activity, and making choices about our personal levels of activity on a day-to-day basis. Sound complicated? It doesn't have to be. Let me introduce you to the simple and inexpensive pedometer. Read on.

The Promise of Pedometers

The idea of using some sort of instrument to count the number of times you step during a day is nothing new. Leonardo DaVinci considered such an instrument in his quest for a distance-measuring device to construct maps both for military purposes and canal construction (12).

The pedometer that Leonardo invented was based on a pendulum's swinging action, possibly inspired by the swing of legs during walking. But his design didn't work well for measuring distances so Leonardo invented a wheelbarrow-like odometer instead. Every few turns of the wheel it dropped a pellet into a box. At the end of the distance traveled, the pellets were counted up and the distance was calculated based on the known circumference of the wheel. We still use the odometer to measure distance (there's one in your car)—although we no longer have to count pellets, of course.

It is foolish to suggest we all start running around pushing wheelbarrows in front of us to determine how far we walk each day. Leonardo's invention was designed to measure distance for purposes of commerce and/or war; it was never intended as a motivational tool for tracking physical activity.

15

Compared with modern times, Leonardo lived in a time characterized by more opportunities to be naturally active—there was no need to track physical activity in his era! But times and circumstances have changed and modern incarnations of the pedometer have evolved to address a new need. Earlier mechanical versions were not dependably accurate and researchers discounted them for the most part. Today a number of commercially available electronic pedometers are considered accurate and reliable. And researchers are slowly beginning to accept their potential for measuring physical activity, specifically ambulatory activity, or walking behavior.

What Pedometers Do and Do Not Measure

Although pedometers have been around for quite awhile, they never quite caught on as personal feedback gadgets.

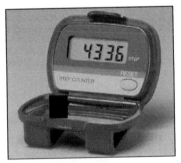

Pedometer. Front view

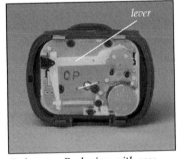

Pedometer. Back view with case removed to show the lever.

One of the reasons, I believe, is a general confusion about what they do and do not accurately measure. I'll cut to the chase: pedometers accurately count steps taken, with less accuracy they can be used to estimate distance walked, and with the least amount of accuracy they can be used to estimate calories burned. I will explain each of these points. The bottom line is that the pedometer is perfect for step counting, which is all you need to practice Manpo-kei.

To help you understand what pedometers do and do not measure, you'll need to know how one works. So figure out how to open up your particular pedometer so that you can examine its inner workings. Likely you will see a lever of sorts that deflects with vertical oscillations (being shaken up-and-down). Each deflection of the lever will register on the pedometer output screen. Now, put it back together and attach the pedometer to your waistband. When you walk your hips move up-and-down—and the pedometer's lever gently shakes up-and-down—with each step you take. The pedometer counts the number of times the lever deflects and outputs the number as steps.

But the pedometer is not perfect. For example, some movements such as weight-shifting, bending, or jumping may deflect the lever and be recorded as a step. In this sense, the term step is a misrepresentation of the movement. It is also true that even the new electronic pedometers are not going to pick up steps taken during slow walking (like those taken while milling around the kitchen preparing dinner). So, your pedometer will count some non-steps as steps and miss some true steps—if you can follow that. But compared to the rest of the day, the relative importance of these errors is likely to be small. From a health promotion perspective, missing steps during slow walking is probably not a problem since we're most interested in measuring activity that is of moderate intensity, such as brisk walking, and the pedometer is very good at capturing that type of activity (13).

Now my argument against estimating distance from the raw step-counts. Some pedometers are equipped to estimate distance based on an average stride-length of some make-believe human being, or the manufacturers may ask you to measure your own stride-length and enter this value into the pedometer's electronic memory. This type of pedometer has been constructed to multiply steps by the entered stride-length to tell you how far you have walked in miles or kilometers. The problem is that distance is horizontal, whereas pedometers detect vertical movement. Extrapolating from a counted step to a horizontal distance requires faith in some constant relationship between the two dimensions that just doesn't exist. Throughout the day your stride lengths will vary—some shorter, some longer. Try this: walk at least a block in one direction, check the pedometer, and walk back the same distance. Although the values should be close, I bet you they won't agree exactly. But don't blame the pedometer—you likely shimmied to the right, swerved a bit, stutter-stepped, dodged a pebble, etc. In other words, you were not able to walk with robot-like consistent stride-lengths—don't worry about it—you're human—it's a skill you can live without.

Similarly, some people have smaller stride-lengths. If such a person takes the same number of steps during the day as someone with a longer stride-length, you might conclude that the first person was less active if you only looked at distance walked! For example, if two individuals each walked 6,500 steps in a single day, but their stride-lengths were 1.6 and 2.4 feet, their distance traveled would be 2.0 and 3.2 miles respectively—a difference of over one mile !

Some pedometers come with the ability to estimate calories burned. This time the manufacturers require that you enter your weight, age, and gender, or some mix of these factors, to calculate energy expenditure based on the number of steps detected. That is because we know that, for the same activity, heavier people burn more calories than lighter people, younger people burn more calories than older people, and men burn more calories than women. Generally, that is. Each time we make an assumption another layer of error is added.

A problem occurs, however, when we try to draw conclusions about activity based on energy expenditure. For example, consider two people who walk step-for-step beside each other during the day, but one is obese and the other is normal weight. At the end of the day, who do you think has burned more calories? Yes, that's right, the obese individual. But if you looked only at their pedometer outputs as calories burned, you might have concluded that the one individual was considerably more active than the other!

The pedometer does not detect intensity of exercise—so if you run, it won't give you credit for how fast or strenuous your workout is. But it will accurately count the number of steps you take. The good news is—you get many more steps running than walking for the same time invested. More bang for the buck so to speak. (I'm not implying that you should take up running. It isn't for everyone. I simply want to point out what the pedometer has to offer those who like to run).

I also need to let you know that pedometers cannot pick up some activities, most obviously swimming (don't take it in the water—it's pointless and your pedometer probably won't work again), bicycling and resistance training (e.g., weight training). Think about these latter two activities. Because you're seated when you ride a bike, a pedometer attached to your waistband won't detect an up-and-down motion of your hips. However, resist the temptation to slip your pedometer into your sock while riding your bike—it won't be counting true steps anyway and you'll probably end up losing it. As for resistance training, it's an activity that has many health benefits. But you'll get no credit from a pedometer for time spent doing dumbbell curls. (So, for time spent in these activities I suggest adding Bonus Steps to your daily count—but you'll learn more about this plan in the chapter called *The Next Step*).

Let me wrap up this section: to practice Manpo-kei, all you need to know is how many steps you take on a daily basis, or steps/day, and a pedometer is very accurate at detecting that. As a personal feedback gadget, the lowest-tech pedometer (i.e., step counter) gives you all you need to know.

Other Motion Sensors

There is another type of motion sensor you might consider: the accelerometer.

Accelerometers are most often used in research although some commercial accelerometers are now available for personal use. They are similar to pedometers in that they sense distortion due to movement of a sensitive lever or series of levers suspended in different planes. Some accelerometers sense both initiation of movement (which might be interpreted as a step) and speed of the movement (which might be interpreted as intensity). Usually these two factors are multiplied and the displayed output is something called activity counts. But speed of movement may not always translate to intensity of movement. Let's say you hike up a mountain, or climb some stairs. You typically decrease your speed of stepping going uphill. The accelerometer detects the slow movement as you climb, interprets it as low intensity, and you don't get full credit for the true intensity of the activity.

Manufacturers of some accelerometers also provide the option of estimating distance traveled (based on stride-length) and energy expended (based on weight, age, and gender information). But as with pedometers, these calculations are likely faulty because they are based on too many assumptions. Accelerometers can probably detect movement during slow walking better than pedometers. But like pedometers they can't pick up swimming or bicycling or give you sufficient credit for weight training. Some accelerometers also require a

21

computer interface and software to download daily activity information (15). In contrast, you won't have to log on anywhere to get immediate feedback using a pedometer—just look down at the display screen. Although the idea of advanced technology may be appealing in this digital age, it makes the accelerometer the more expensive and inconvenient option. In comparison to accelerometers ($50-$450 + requisite add-ons), pedometers are cheap ($20-$60). And you won't cry as much if you accidentally drop one down the toilet.

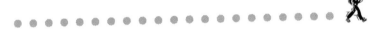

The Japanese Experience

The Japanese experience, the "10,000 Steps/day" Slogan, and the Rebirth of Manpo-kei.

When it comes to using a simple pedometer to track and increase steps/day, the Japanese are way ahead of us. A Japanese company manufactured a version of the pedometer in 1965 and nicknamed it "Manpo-kei," which literally translates to "10,000 steps meter" (16). Walking and hiking organizations adopted and promoted the goal as a slogan and the Japanese public loved it. Today in Japan most people are aware of the slogan and pedometers are common household items.

Unfortunately for English-speaking societies, the early scientific literature supporting the use of the pedometer as a tracking and motivational tool was published primarily in Japanese. Without translation, the contents of these articles were inaccessible to most North American researchers and health-care workers. Lucky for us, Japanese researchers began publishing their pedometer studies in English-language journals. One notable Japanese study was published in 1996 comparing two groups of obese and sedentary men with type 2 diabetes (17).

Both groups lived in a hospital and were given a special diet. Only one group was told to take at least 10,000 steps/day using a pedometer. The pedometer-program group averaged 19,200 steps/day and at the end of the 6-8 week study lost an average of 17 lb. (almost 8 lbs. more than the second group that dieted only and averaged 4,500 steps/day). Dramatic results such as these make researchers take notice. Many have been inspired to reconsider the simple and inexpensive pedometer, particularly for its motivational value.

I'm one of those inspired researchers. Researchers, including me, have consistently reported an inverse relationship between pedometer steps/day and measures of body fatness; the more overweight/obese people are, the fewer steps they take (18-21). In one study of over 100 people (18), I found those with values greater than approximately 9,000 steps/day were more frequently classified as normal weight. On the other hand, people with values less than approximately 5,000 steps/day were more frequently classified as obese. I found similar cut points in another study of 160 individuals with type 2 diabetes (22).

But I'm reluctant to proclaim that everyone needs to achieve 10,000 steps/day for health. Let me tell you why. While it is tempting to jump in and go with a simple slogan, in my opinion there isn't sufficient scientific evidence at this time to support it. But wait, you say, what about the Japanese study I just described?! True, the men were told to take 10,000 steps/day. But if you look closely, you'll see that the men who benefited from the program took 19,200 steps/day. So this study doesn't really tell us about the benefits of walking 10,000 steps/day. Some North American experts suggest that 15,000 steps/day is a more appropriate goal for weight loss and maintenance (23).

To tell the truth, I'm hesitant to generalize any specific number of steps/day based on the results of the Japanese 10,000 steps/day study. Generalizability has to do with how confident a researcher is in extending conclusions about the findings of one small study to all people everywhere. Motivation plays a major role in achieving and maintaining activity goals. In the Japanese study, the men lived in a hospital and were likely surrounded by supportive and encouraging staff members 24-hours a day. This is an artificial lifestyle, so the results might be difficult to reproduce in the everyday world of the average North American. The level of support those men enjoyed is rare outside a hospital or spa-like setting.

Accumulating research does tell us that 10,000 steps/day seems to be a reasonable Baseline Level (usual steps/day level before behavior change) for young and/or apparently healthy individuals but it may be too low for children (as you will see in the next chapter). And it is unreasonably high for sedentary populations, particularly those comprised of older individuals and persons with chronic health problems like arthritis, diabetes, and heart disease (14). If a goal is unreasonable it will be difficult to sustain. A recent study of middle-aged workers reported that of 730 people who began a 10,000 steps/day program, only 83 could keep it up for 12 weeks (24)!

Regardless of the actual value, promoting any single rigid number of steps/day as a universal goal implies that no benefits occur below that level and we don't know that yet either. I do know that many of the folks I've worked with have reaped benefits (e.g., weight loss, reduced waist girth, enhanced fitness, improved blood pressure) from substantially increasing their steps/day using the pedometer (sometimes doubling their steps/day). But those same folks found the magical number of 10,000 steps/day impossible to reach. The key to health benefits doesn't seem to be about achieving some arbitrary number of steps/day—it's more about increasing your personal number of steps/day relative to your own individual Baseline Level, or what I call More Than Before. Let me explain using our heroine Susan as an example. If Susan averages 2,000 steps/day before beginning Manpo-kei, then she increases it to 8,000 steps/day—that's a four-fold increase in physical activity (excellent, amazing, truly outstanding are descriptors that come to mind)—but still shy of the Japanese health slogan. I am concerned that Susan (or anyone else like her) might interpret her effort as a shortfall compared to the 10,000 steps/day arbitrary goal, become frustrated and give up. Viewed from a Baseline Level of 2,000 steps/day, 10,000 or 15,000 steps/day may seem insurmountable (trust me, it's a huge jump, as I will illustrate in the next chapter). If Susan (or anyone else) just ends up giving up, no divinely inspired goal is worth the price of the paper it's written on.

Let me emphasize this again: it all depends on your Baseline Level. For example, if you discover your average is 15,000 steps/day at baseline and your desire is to lose weight, obviously 10,000 steps/day is a ridiculous goal and 15,000 steps/day isn't going to change a thing either. At this point you will need to decide whether you want to increase your steps/day or refine your eating behaviors (or both) to create an energy deficit (but more on this later).

After carefully considering all the evidence, I have come to the conclusion that there needs to be a trade-off between effectiveness and sustainability. Somewhere, for each individual, there exists some goal that: 1) represents an improvement over Baseline (More Than Before); and, 2) can be reasonably sustained over the long-term. That's why I propose a more individualized way to practice Manpo-kei. You will learn that the Manpo-kei philosophy I advocate moves beyond promoting a single universal slogan. In my version, the Manpo-kei concept is reborn to represent the personal art and science of step counting to reclaim natural physical activity. From here on, I will use Manpo-kei to mean an individualized approach to increasing physical activity through a pedometer-based program of goal-setting and self-monitoring.

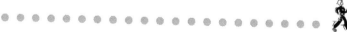

How Many Steps Do People Take?

How many steps do people take and how do they do it?

By now you are probably sitting at the edge of your seat and asking, "So, how many steps should I take?" Good question. The answer for now is: More Than Before. But before you proceed, I want to give you more information to help you relate to the step data that you will eventually generate when you practice Manpo-kei.

I'm often asked how many steps people take on average. This type of information is called normative data or expected values. Expected values will help you get a feel for how many steps different people take in different situations and what you might anticipate when you first wear your pedometer. I've pieced this step data together from a number of studies conducted with a variety of people. Expected values for steps/day are: between 12,000 and 16,000 steps/day for 8-10 year old children (lower for girls than boys); between 7,000-13,000 steps/day for relatively healthy, younger (20-40 years) adults (lower for women than men); between 6,000-8,500 steps/day for healthy older (50-

70 years) adults; and between 3,500-5,500 steps/day for adults living with disabilities and chronic illnesses (14).

I've also read some studies that report steps/day for people from different occupations (16,25). Combined with my own experience in collecting pedometer data, I can reasonably say that if you work in a job that is mostly sitting, say, telephone operator or office worker, you may get 4,000-5,000 steps/day. If you are on your feet all day at work, but not really walking about (like a pharmacist or hairstylist), then you may get 5,500-6,500 steps/day. If you are frequently on the move at work, say, a nurse, waiter/waitress, you can fluctuate between 8,000-20,000 steps/day. Regardless of what you do to pay the bills, when Sunday rolls around and you don't work you may get only 2,000-3,000 steps. If you take a holiday from work, say, a trip to Rome, and enjoy a day of sightseeing you might reach 30,000 steps! And I know from personal experience that on days when I stay home from work because I'm sick, I'm lucky if I get 500 steps/day!

These expected values are loose guidelines to be interpreted cautiously. Personal circumstances differ wildly and very few individuals will fit a cookie-cutter approach to predicting steps/day based only on gender, age, or occupation. You actually have quite a bit of control over how many steps you accumulate on a daily basis. Manpo-kei allows you to evaluate your Baseline within the context of your unique life situation. From this position you will be able to make important personal choices and regain control of your naturally active lifestyle. Let me show you how it all comes together by describing a Manpo-kei Make-over.

Manpo-kei Make-over

A Manpo-kei Make-over describes simple lifestyle changes that result in dramatic increases in steps/day.

Think back to the scenario I presented in the chapter called *The Evolution of Physical Inactivity*. You remember our heroine, Susan, whose only physical activity during the day was a 20-minute walk on the treadmill? She was an office worker. If she had worn a pedometer that day, she would have registered between 4,000-5,000 steps. Her daily routine offered little opportunity to accumulate incidental steps outside the intentional steps she took during her scheduled exercise sessions. If that routine continued, day after day, she would have trouble keeping her weight down, even though she intentionally exercised at a fitness club! So how could Susan improve the situation? Let me create a Manpo-kei version of the same scenario.

Susan begins the morning by hitting the snooze button to extend her repose but eventually gives in and gets up. She showers, dresses and clips on her pedometer. The whole family is wearing them now. Her husband takes the dog for a walk around the block. It's Susan's morning to meet the neighborhood kids on the corner and walk them six blocks to school (the parents on her block take turns)(26). Susan looks forward to this opportunity to banter with her kids' friends and catch up with their hectic lives. A block from the school, her husband picks her up (avoiding the anxious-parent traffic-jam) and drives her to the train. On her way into the city, Susan catches up on her reading, and then enjoys the short walk to her office building, stopping by the bank machine and then the local coffee vendor for one "to go." At work she chooses to take the stairs to the second floor before settling into her cubicle. Mid-morning, while considering a pressing project, she walks downstairs to the outside courtyard for a brief stroll. Back inside she resumes work with renewed fervor. At lunch, Susan and an officemate walk to one of their favorite lunch spots. In the afternoon she has to spend quite a bit of time speaking with clients on the phone. She is thankful hers is a cordless so she can pace to wear off some frustration that builds up from time-to-time. After work Susan walks to the train and heads home. Her husband picks her up at the station. The kids have stayed later at school for a soccer game and are walking home with some older neighborhood kids. Susan and her husband swing by the video store to select the evening's entertainment. She is no longer annoyed about how far she has to park from the door since it means a few extra steps on her pedometer and a little closer to her Step Goal! At home Susan slips into her running gear and goes for a 20-minute brisk walk/jog with her neighbor from down the street. Susan has been doing this for awhile and both she and her husband are thinking about running a 5K race later in the year. He does his running on his lunch break because there are shower facilities at his workplace. Susan arrives home to find the kids playing in the backyard while her husband finishes the lawn with his pushmower. Inside, she wonders how anyone could have lived without microwaves, dishwashers, and washers and dryers. Dinner is served in front of the TV—everyone crowds around the couch for the video (some things never change). After the flick the whole family takes the dog for a walk around the block. Before Susan goes to bed she checks her pedometer and writes the results in her Tracking Calendar: 15, 675 steps—well above her Step Goal. Her husband has 17,367—he ran a couple of extra errands. Their kids each have 16,452 and 21,456 steps. The one with the highest steps today played basketball in physical education class and went on a field trip to a museum. The routine plays out much the same way, week after week. A month later Susan notices her pants are fitting a little looser, her husband looks more handsome, and her kids aren't quite as roly-poly. Something good is happening. Manpo-kei.

By making some simple lifestyle-changes Susan was able to triple her steps/day from 5,000 to 15,000! I use this Manpo-kei Make-over story as an example of how anyone can increase their steps/day by changing some simple daily routines. Everyone's daily life differs somewhat and therefore not everyone will have the same goals or use the same strategies to reach these goals. That's why I recommend a more individualized approach to counting and increasing your steps/day.

Practicing Manpo-kei

Go for simplicity. Get a pedometer that offers the fewest buttons. All you need is something that counts steps.

Choosing the Pedometer for You

Let's assume you're ready to start stepping. You'll need a pedometer. There are a number of commercial brands available, and if this idea catches on, I predict that in a very short time there will be even more of a selection available to you! I don't feel right about endorsing any specific brand, but I will give you some tips that will help you decide which pedometer is right for you.

These are the primary characteristics I look for when buying a pedometer (there is a Shopping Checklist in Appendix A). It must be small, lightweight, have an extended battery life (expect at least 3 years), have an easy-to-read digital step-counter display, have a secure attachment-clip, the fewer buttons the better (and those buttons should not be too easily reset with just normal bumping and banging around), and, it must be cheap. It must of course be accurate. Now I will go into more detail on each point.

Manpo-kei can be a silent art if you want it to be. If that is the case, then you want a pedometer to be small and lightweight. You are the only one who needs to know you're wearing it. For the utmost in private self-monitoring consider wearing it so it faces into your body instead of facing the world. And if you don't have a waistband (e.g., you're wearing some sort of overalls or a dress without a waistband) attach it to your underwear! If private self-monitoring is not for you, you can wear it more obviously as a conversation piece—people are bound to ask you about it if they see it!

An extended battery life is a given. You want it to keep working for a long time without having to worry about it. Expect the same battery life as you would from your watch—pedometers usually run off that same type of battery. The digital display monitor should be easy to read and stand up to long-term wear and tear (numbers should not fade over time).

The quality of the attachment-clip is important. Pedometers need to stay on securely, or you'll get most of your increased activity chasing after them and picking them up. The attachment-clip should have some sort of ribbing or otherwise knurled surface that comes into contact with your waistband—if the clip is too smooth it is apt to fly off during bending movements, especially if you carry a little extra weight around your belly. The other thing about the attachment-clip you need to know and respect is how flexible it is. If the clip is quite rigid, it might break off if you try to wedge it over a combination of clothing and a leather belt—and then the pedometer is useless of course. If the pedometer doesn't come with an idiot-string (a security string attaching the pedometer to your clothing), consider making one yourself using a string and a safety pin. Just tie the string to the pedometer clip and slide the safety pin through the free end of the string. Then pin it to your waistband. More than one person I've worked with (okay, me too) can relate stories of near misses (or direct hits) with the toilet bowl. Let me tell you right now: always keep an eye on your pedometer when you're in the bathroom—you'll thank me for this tip someday.

Go for simplicity. Get a pedometer that offers the fewest buttons. All you need is something that counts steps (for the reasons I stated earlier, I don't recommend converting steps to distance traveled or calories expended). The only button you need is a reset button to zero the instrument before you begin accumulating a new day's worth of steps. Don't pay for anything you don't need. But do make sure the pedometer you choose is not too easily reset with just normal everyday movements. It is so disappointing to discover your pedometer reset itself to zero when you put your car seatbelt on at the end of the work day—and you hadn't checked it since before you went for that epic noon-hour walk! Some pedometers come with plastic covers to protect the reset button from just such mishaps.

Accuracy has to do with correctly counting the steps you take. No pedometer I know is perfect, so there will always be a degree of error throughout the day. Remember that some movements like bending, jumping, shifting, might be picked up and counted as a step. But hey, you were moving, right? This is error you can live with. And some slow steps might not be counted at all—but you really only want to count the good ones anyway. This is also error you can live with. So, how can you tell if your pedometer is making errors you can't live with?

You can give the instrument you are considering a quick in-store Pedometer Accuracy Test. If it fails this test, think about buying a different one. Here's the test. Put the pedometer on as the manufacturer suggests (usually clipped to the clothing at your waist, centered over your dominant foot). Make sure it is at zero. Walk at your normal pace and count 20 steps. Look at the pedometer. If it does not say exactly 20 steps, get suspicious. But before you consider it a dud, check its placement. To work, pedometers need to be in a vertical (up-and-down) position. If your pants, or belt, or belly hang on you so that the pedometer is the least bit rotated horizontally (rolled onto its side) it won't give you an accurate reading. Shift the unit around on your waistband until it is absolutely vertical. Then repeat the test. Shift it one more time if you need to. Try the test one last time. If it continues to be wildly out on the count, the unit may be a dud. Do not buy. Approach the process like you would for buying running shoes—try the pedometer on— test it out—fiddle with its placement—see if it works for you before buying.

Let's talk money. As long as the above needs are met, go cheap. Expect to pay between $20 and $60. Unless you have a fail-proof idiot-string, you may lose the occasional pedometer. It is a lot easier to get over the loss of a $20 pedometer than a $60 one.

Once you have purchased your pedometer, you will need to establish your Baseline Level. Read on.

● ●

Getting a Baseline

It is important to know how many steps you usually take in a day now before you start practicing Manpo-kei.

It's like knowing how much you weigh before going on a diet— it helps you track your progress and determine your success. Just for fun, try to guess how many steps you take considering what I've already told you in the chapter called *How Many Steps Do People Take ?*

Write your estimate down here:

- -

and look at it again after you've finished the next task.

For one week, live your life as usual. Just wear the pedometer during your waking hours (take it off if you bathe or swim) and record the day-end value in the Baseline Activity Calendar located in Appendix B. Circle Y=Yes or N=No to record whether you worked that day, or if you participated in sport or exercise. If you did any sport or exercise, record the time and type of activity in just a few words (e.g., "soccer 30 minutes", or "walk for exercise 15 minutes"). Remember that exercise is intentional activity done for its own sake, so don't worry about recording all other incidental walking you do during the day—that is your pedometer's job. Completing this calendar each day should take you less than a minute. After this first week you won't have to include this much detail unless you want to. Every morning make sure to reset the pedometer to zero before you begin accumulating a new day's worth of steps. Starting with a blank pedometer every day will allow you to look at the results from each day of the week separately and draw conclusions about your habits. To make sure you are really capturing your typical activities, try not to look at the pedometer at all until the end of the day. This first week of self-monitoring without changing your behavior is very important to understanding your habits more fully.

At the end of the week, use the Baseline Activity Worksheet (Appendix C) to calculate your average steps/day. This is your Baseline Level. Then to help you understand how your lifestyle contributes to your steps/day, determine how many steps you average on your workdays, on days off (e.g., weekends), on days you exercise or do sport, on days when you don't do exercise or sport, etc.

The next part of this chapter is designed as an interactive workbook. So get out your pencil and consider the following:

How close was your guess (look back at page 39) Were there any surprises?

How does your Baseline Level compare with the expected values for different age and occupational groups I described on pages 29-30.

Generally, if you average lower than 5,000 steps/day, you have a lot to gain by increasing your steps/day. If you average between 5,000 and 9,000 steps/day you could benefit from increasing your physical activity. If you average between 9,000-13,000 steps/day, you are reasonably active now, but you could still benefit from continued self-monitoring and engagement in a variety of intentional moderate- to vigorous-intensity activities. And if you average over 13,000 steps/day, you are likely already engaged in intentional activities, including sport and exercise. You might choose to wear a pedometer to maintain consistently high steps.

Look closely now at your patterns of activity. Answer the following list of questions:

What days are highest?

_____

_____

What days are lowest?

_____

_____

What are the specific days of the week when you are highest/lowest *(is it Monday and Wednesday? Tuesday and Saturday? Workdays? Exercise days? Weekend days or other days off? Holidays?)*

_____

_____

Once you have identified your personal patterns of activity—try to explain them in terms of your behaviors. Let me help you get started.

Think back to the specific behaviors and try to explain the number of steps on your highest days. Did you walk to work? Did you run errands? Did you go shopping? Did you take in a special event in your community? Did you go sight-seeing? Write your answers down:

_____

Now, what did you do differently on the days when your steps were lowest? Did you travel by car for a long time? Did you work at your computer a lot? Did you play video games? Did you sit around a lot? Did you watch a lot of TV? Explain your lowest days:

Summarize: what are the specific activities that give you the most number of steps? Now realistically consider—can you do more of these activities?

What are the activities that register few or no steps? Again, realistically consider—can you do fewer of these activities?

There are no right or wrong answers—each person is apt to create a slightly different list. You need to consider what is realistic for you. What are you willing to add to your life? And what are you unwilling to give up?

• •

Decision-Balance Process ....

Let me guide you through a decision-balance process designed to help you weigh the pros and cons of the behavior change you're considering.

Aﬅer the process of monitoring and reﬂecting you should be much more aware of your lifestyle and the number of steps you take each day. Now you need to decide what action to take, if any. Let me guide you through a decision-balance process designed to help you weigh the pros and cons of the behavior change you're considering (27,28). Once again, I'm going to give you some questions to reﬂect on before beginning a program of increasing your steps/day. So keep your pencil handy.

If you become more active (e.g., take more steps/day), what personal benefits do you think you will get? I've already listed several benefits elsewhere in this book, but think about your personal circumstance. Make a list of what you personally believe you will gain. For example, one woman I worked with believed that increasing her steps/day would allow her to prepare for her upcoming trip to Disneyland with her grandchildren, something that would normally wear her out! So now it's your turn—write down what benefits you believe you will get from becoming more active:

_____

_____

No behavior change comes without some trade-off. So now consider what you will have to give up if you become more active. It may not seem obvious right now, but think about giving up some time watching TV, driving in the car, taking elevators, etc. How much are these behaviors worth to you? How many of these could you realistically give up? What can't you live without? One couple I worked with said they absolutely could not give up their TV-watching time together. Face these realities now so you can make some informed decisions later. Once again, write down what you'll have to give up if you become more active:

And it is not just yourself you have to think about. Your behaviors have an impact on those you live and work with on a day-to-day basis. You must also consider what gains and losses they might experience if you pursue an increased number of steps/day. Again think about your personal circumstance. Who depends on you, and what do they depend on you for? What impact might your lifestyle-change have on them?

Once you have this all laid out in front of you, you will need to do some problem-solving before you get into setting any goals. What can you do to maximize the gains, to yourself and others, and minimize the losses? Can you kill two birds with any single stones? For example, one of the women I worked with worried that she might end up giving up time with her young son if she pursued what she believed to be self-centered leisure time activities. So she began walking to her son's school to walk him home at the end of the schoolday. In this way she was able to increase her steps/day and spend more time with her child. A factory foreman found that he could increase his steps/day by getting out of the office and onto the factory floor everyday, twice a day. An unanticipated effect of this simple strategy was an improved rapport with his co-workers. And remember the couple with the TV-watching addiction? Well, they dusted off their neglected treadmill and took turns watching and walking.

No behavior change is easy. And although it seems simple, increasing your steps/day is the result of a conscious behavior change that will not only have an impact on you but on the ones who live out their lives beside you. Taking time to consider the full impact of any behavior change can help you make choices that will lead to your success.

● ●

Goal -Setting

Goal-setting is a process of identifying a desired state or behavior that you can work towards.

Goal-setting is common to health, business, the arts, academics, etc. Universally, however, the appropriateness of a goal is evaluated using a simple acronym: SMART, that is it must be Specific, Measurable, Attainable, Realistic, and Time-limited (or have an identifiable Time-frame). Using pedometers to count steps/day can be very SMART. You choose a Specific value for increasing your steps/day that is also Measurable using your pedometer. In Manpo-kei, the daily goal you set is called a Step Goal—or a number of steps you want to attain by the end of the day. Having spent time reflecting on your habits and completing the decision-balance process, you are ready to set an Attainable and Realtistic Step Goal. And the Time-frame is simple: a day. The beauty of Manpo-kei is that each day represents a new attempt at your Step Goal. Each day stands alone. Each day you reset your pedometer and start again, regardless of what the previous day's result was. Of course, a string of seven days is a week, and you can also evaluate your progress on a weekly basis. I'll show you how.

First, let's figure out how many steps you take in 10 minutes of continuous walking. So, put the book down, reset your pedometer to zero, check the time on your watch, and walk at your normal pace for 10 minutes. How many steps do you take in 10 minutes?

Earlier I mentioned that public health recommendations say you should accumulate 30 minutes of moderate activity, like brisk walking, on most, if not all days of the week. To find out how many steps you take in 30 minutes just multiply the above value by 3:

You might decide to add this number to your Baseline Level to set a Step Goal. Any number of steps you add to your Baseline Level is called a Step Increment. Just for fun add the Step Increment (equivalent to 30 minutes of walking) to your Baseline Level:

Study this new number. How does it measure up as a Step Goal? It is definitely Specific and Measurable. And if you make it a daily goal the Time-frame is clear. The big questions you need to consider are: 1) Is it Attainable; and, 2) Is it Realistic? Having monitored your typical activities for a week, you should have a good idea whether it's the right Step Goal for you. Here's a tip: you should be at least 80% confident that you can make your Step Goal on a daily basis for one full week. If you feel anything less than 80% confident, adjust your Step Goal to a level you feel better about.

No one can set this Step Goal for you. This is part of the individualized process of Manpo-kei. This is your choice. Just aim for More Than Before. What's the worst thing that can happen? You discover your Step Goal isn't really that SMART. It's a learning process. As a practitioner of Manpo-kei you get to reassess and reset your Step Goal every week. So, right now, choose a personal Step Increment you can add to your Baseline Level that gives you a Step Goal you think you can reach for at least seven days.

Baseline Level + Step Increment = Step Goal

You now have a SMART Manpo-kei Step Goal for your first week that is also More Than Before.

● ●

Strategies

Strategies are the behaviors you practice to meet your Step Goal every day.

In addition to goals you need strategies. Strategies are the behaviors you practice to meet your Step Goal every day. Remember when you were monitoring yourself for your Baseline Level? I told you to go about your typical day and try not to look at the pedometer until the end of the day. Well, that rule no longer stands. In fact, one universal strategy I recommend is to look at your pedometer frequently throughout the day. Keep in mind your Step Goal and steadily work towards it as you live out your day. If by noon you don't have many steps accumulated, you may have to consider additional afternoon or evening activities to make your Step Goal. You can also refer to the pedometer regularly throughout the day for general feedback about the impact your habits have on your natural activity levels. What is it that you do that increases or decreases your step totals? You will be able to use this information to refine both your Step Goal and strategies.

Other strategies are more individualized and reflect your own lifestyle, preferences, and schedules. These are some of the strategies used by people I've worked with: park farther from the office entrance, take the stairs (up and/or down) instead of elevators, walk to lunch, take the dog for a walk, go for a walk in the evenings with your spouse, leave the car at home and walk to the convenience store. Hopefully, these examples have inspired you to think about simple strategies that reflect your own unique lifestyle. At this point in the program, however, I recommend you narrow it down to a single strategy—something you are comfortable with trying for one week. Over the next few weeks you will have opportunities to experiment with a variety of strategies. For now write down one personal strategy that you will try for this next week:

● ●

Tracking

Experts know that tracking, or self-monitoring, is crucial to the success of any planned behavior change (27). Tracking your daily steps in relation to your Step Goal is important feedback on your progress, helping you to identify patterns (i.e., successes and rough spots) and refine strategies. Fortunately, tracking is simple using a pedometer and calendar combination. The pedometer tracks your daily activity and the calendar tracks your long-term activity. So, in anticipation of beginning your Manpo-kei program, write down your Step Goal in the appropriate spot on the Tracking Calendar provided in Appendix D. Notice that this calendar is simpler to complete than the Baseline Activity Calendar. It is intended for long-term tracking—how long is up to you, but you should try to commit to at least four weeks of tracking initially (writing it down each night), and then from time to time thereafter as a Booster Shot (a process of re-assessment and re-commitment to Step Goals). I'll give you a four-week Tracking Calendar to begin with, but any calendar will do once you get into the habit. Tomorrow the fun of Manpo-kei begins.

Today is the First Day of the Rest of Your Life!

When you wake up and get dressed, reset your pedometer to zero and clip it on. Remember to look at your pedometer frequently and practice your selected strategy as you work towards your Step Goal. Tonight and each night before you go to bed, write down your day-end total of steps in the Tracking Calendar. Take a moment to compare it to the Step Goal you set for yourself. If you have met the Step Goal for that day, circle Y=Yes, otherwise circle N=No. If not, rest assured that tomorrow is a new day and a new beginning to the rest of your life. Renew your commitment. You'll be going into each new day powered with even more knowledge about yourself and what it means to be naturally physically active. This is the Manpo-kei way.

● ●

Reflection & Refinement

Manpo-kei is characterized by a continual process of goal reflection and refinement.

Keep stepping and tracking for a string of seven days—one week. Determine your average Steps/day, or—your Current Steps/day (which replaces your Baseline Level and reflects this week's accomplishment), by totaling steps taken for the whole week and dividing by 7. In addition, count up the number of days out of seven that you attained your Step Goal. Now it's time for reflection on your experiences and refinement of your Step Goal. So, once again, I urge you to put pencil to paper and consider the following questions:

Compare your Current Steps/day to your Baseline Level. Then compare it to your Step Goal. How did you do—are you doing More Than Before?

If you didn't quite meet your Step Goal but you did increase over and above your Baseline Level, it might suggest that your goal was a little unrealistic at this time. On the other hand, you might discover that your Current Steps/day is higher than your Step Goal —which may mean you're actually capable of doing more steps/day and your original goal was not challenging enough!

Now let's consider the number of days that you achieved your Step Goal. If you are trying to meet the public health recommendations for minimal activity, you need to reach your Step Goal on most, if not all days. That means 5 to 7 days a week. How do you compare to this benchmark?

If you reached your Step Goal at least 5-7 days last week, great going! However, if you found it too easy to attain, you might consider increasing your Step Goal. If you did not meet your Step Goal at least 5 days a week, consider readjusting your Step Goal to make it more Realistic for you at this time.

Before you redefine your Step Goal for a new week, assess the success of your selected strategy. Did it work for you? Why or why not?

Did other strategies emerge during the week that worked out better for you? Describe these:

Your answers will help you decide if you need to consider other strategies as you work towards your Step Goal. Since you are still relatively new to Manpo-kei, you may need to play with different strategies. Remember it is not only what you do but also what you don't do. Consider strategies that will help increase steps (e.g., walk to the post office, self-caddy a golf game), but also consider those that might help reduce inactivity. Shorten periods of time when you accumulate no steps or very few steps at all (e.g., video-tape favorite shows to regulate time spent watching TV, reduce time spent in the car by avoiding drive-through windows). It only takes a few weeks of practicing Manpo-kei to discover which strategies really work for you and which ones don't.

This next question also relates to your selection of strategies, and the answer to it is vitally important to your success. Who did you show your pedometer to—and what was their response?

It's not a stupid question. We know that social support—from friends, family, co-workers, and others—is extremely important to beginning and sustaining any sort of behavior change (28). And this is true for any type of physical activity behavior change, including one that uses pedometers! Who are the people around you who have the power to influence the number of steps you take during the day—either positively or negatively?

What can these people do for you to help you meet your Step Goal?

Now plan some time to talk with them about it (perhaps during a walk).[1]

---

[1] *You will likely find that most people will want to borrow your pedometer and find out how many steps they take! But this pedometer is a personal gadget for your use—it will only work for you if you wear it. Suggest your friends and family take a walk beside you and you will tell them the number of steps you took during the walk! Otherwise, get them their own pedometer.*

So now that you've answered a few more questions, it's time to commit once again, in writing. People tell me it's easier to do this the second week because they know more about themselves and which strategies do or do not work for them. So now, write down your Current Steps/day for this first week, choose a Step Increment in the same way you did last week, and add the two together to get next week's new Step Goal. Make sure that the new Step Goal is SMART and that you are at least 80% confident that you can attain this new Step Goal on a daily basis, for one full week.

Current Steps/day + Step Increment = Step Goal

Don't be afraid of the number you end up with. Remember what you actually accomplished last week! And let me reassure you in case you're panicking about having to increase your Step Goal every week. Somewhere in the next couple of weeks, you will discover a SMART and sustainable Step Goal. Most of the folks I've worked with found it within only four weeks of practice and self-monitoring. Believe me, at some point you'll say, "This level is right for me in my life." And that level will likely be well above your Baseline Level, or More Than Before.

But before you rush off to begin a new week of accumulating steps, consider your strategies once again. This time write down two strategies. And I'll even let you keep the one from the week before if it worked for you:

So that's it. You have a new Step Goal and new strategies (or you are keeping the ones that work), including engaging the people who live out their lives beside you. Every week, re-calculate your Current Steps/day and determine how many days you actually achieved your Step Goal. Then re-read this section on Reflection and Refinement. Answering all the questions again will guide you in determining how you did in relation to your Step Goal and which strategies worked (and which ones didn't). Finally, set another Step Goal and select strategies for the next week. Manpo-kei is meant to be a simple and repetitive art! Enjoy the process—it really is quite entertaining and can be the topic of many conversations!

● ●

What to Watch Out For

It is true what they say about people being creatures of habit.

Just think of any behavior you've tried to change— smoking, dieting, exercising, mailing off birthday cards on time (my own personal failing), etc. It's not easy. We keep falling back into our old, comfortable habits. And when we fall back we too easily lose our motivation, become discouraged, and want to give up.

That's why it's important to recognize high-risk situations and plan for a relapse. A high-risk situation is one you recognize as potentially leading to a backslide in behavior. For example, 'Must See TV' makes the couch appear a temptress during the long, dark winter months. And of course, a few days of lousy weather makes it difficult to keep to a self-determined mandate to walk at lunch. If high-risk situations such as these lead to inactivity as the rule rather than the exception, then you need a damage-control plan. So, what are the high-risk situations you need to consider? Specifically, what conspires in your life to thwart your goal attempts—and ultimately drives your steps/day down?

Fortunately, wearing a pedometer can help you identify and keep track of unacceptably low activity days. You need to come up with your own unique Lowest Acceptable Level—a number of steps/day that is your personal Inactivity Index. For some people, this is their Baseline Level. Once you have been wearing a pedometer for at least four weeks, decide on a value of steps/day that you think is your Lowest Acceptable Level. Write it down here:

_____

If your day-end total is lower than your Lowest Acceptable Level only every now and then it's not a big deal. But when more and more days of the week are lower than your Lowest Acceptable Level, it's an indication of potential relapse. I suggest a 3-day rule of thumb to define relapse: three or more days of the week below your Lowest Acceptable Level and it's time to renew your commitment and revitalize your strategies.

What can you do to plan for high-risk situations and prevent a relapse? For example, over holidays and special occasions there are usually plenty of opportunities for feasting combined with low activity socializing. Definitely a recipe for low average steps/day. Given such high-risk situations, which strategies can you practice to minimize their impact? Obviously, you can get your steps in earlier in the day in anticipation of the event. Another approach is to take more steps on the other days of the week to make up for a single low day. What are your realistic strategies for dealing with your own high-risk situations?

Practicing these strategies is the only sure-fire way to determine if they work. So, subject yourself to one of your high-risk situations—let your behaviors result in daily steps lower than your Lowest Acceptable Level—and deal with it so it doesn't take over and lead to a relapse. Yes, I'm saying—challenge yourself to successive days of inactivity—then counter its impact in your own unique way.

Another thing to watch out for: attaining high steps/day is not a license to consume large quantities of food, even if said food is low in fat! Be prepared to come to terms with reality. If you document a dramatic and consistent increase in steps/day, and the weight scales don't budge after a month, you need to consider changing your eating behaviors too. For that you'll need another book, and there are plenty of good books on that topic. Whether you want to reduce your weight or not, it's a good idea to have variety and balance in your choice of nutrient-dense foods, moderation in indulgences, and importantly—portion control. No one really needs a second helping and monster-sizing (or whatever the restaurant calls it) is likely to become a self-fulfilling prophecy.

● ●

What to Expect

Although Manpo-kei is simple, it's not a quick fix for years of inactivity.

You must find a level of steps/day that you can sustain over the long haul. Typically I see folks experience a dramatic increase on the order of 2,000-4,000 steps/day when they first start the program. Like those who have stepped before you, you'll likely have some ups and downs until you discover a sustainable level. This level is usually well above your Baseline Level. Do not despair about infrequent days of lower total steps; the secret to Manpo-kei is consistency, or achieving your Step Goal frequently—on most, if not all days of the week.

You can anticipate that self-monitoring using a pedometer is both motivating and enjoyable. Time and time again, I have heard people I work with remark that they are as attached (emotionally) to their pedometers as their pedometers are to them (physically). Some Manpo-kei practitioners speak of their pedometers as if they have distinct personalities and genders! And there is great joy in spotting someone else with a pedometer on and initiating animated conversations comparing strategies and Step Goals. Examples of comments reflecting individual experiences are as follows:

I never realized how inactive I was before I started looking at (the pedometer values) and thinking, holy, I did not do very much—now I make a real effort to get out there and walk.

Every time you think about it, you look at your numbers. You say, "Oh my numbers are low." You got to get out there and do it. Without that pedometer I know that I would not have pushed myself as much.

(The weekly goal-setting) pushed you further every week to do a little bit more—after you do it one or two times you understand what exactly you can do— I found it easier to make small improvements.

You had your bad days and your good days and you could look and see if you were behind. It is right there in front of you all the time. Every morning you look at (the calendar)—it was gratifying.

The more people you told the more people you had helping you—sort of pushing you—not literally but invisibly behind you—sort of cheering you on—I think that's more of a big deal because you told them.

In summary, Manpo-kei is an enjoyable process. Although you may experience some ups and downs as you experiment with setting your Step Goals and strategies, expect personal discovery and growth, a harmless attachment to your personal pedometer, and a feeling of belonging as you receive support from other Manpo-kei converts.

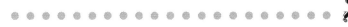

Manpo-kei

The Next Step

If you've worked up to 9,000-13,000 steps/day or more (or your Baseline Level was already this high or higher) and you're interested in reaping further health and fitness benefits from Manpo-kei, this chapter is for you.

I still recommend pedometer self-monitoring because it helps you sort out the factors that sustain your high levels of daily physical activity. I wear a pedometer every day (I believe in practicing what I preach), but I don't think such conduct is necessary for everyone. One woman I worked with decided (after two months of self-monitoring) that she didn't need to wear her pedometer every day. She had developed a strong sense of what she needed to do to be naturally physically active enough to get the health benefits she desired. If you reach a similar level of heightened awareness you may also decide not to wear your pedometer every day. I do recommend, however, that every three months (i.e., at least once a season) you put the pedometer back on. Wear it for a week or two to make sure you're not slipping back into your old habits. Specifically, compare your Current Steps/day to your Baseline Level. Make your decisions based on what you notice: are your Current Steps/day More Than Before—that is, are they higher, lower, or the same as your Baseline Level? Is this acceptable? If not, you may want to return to the goal-setting, self-monitoring, and reflecting cycle for at least four weeks. This process of re-assessing and re-committing to Step Goals is called a Booster Shot.

I want to emphasize that using a pedometer to increase and monitor physical activity does not dismiss the concept of exercise, that is, intentional activity for its own sake. Instead, Manpo-kei recognizes exercise as one of the many strategies you can choose to attain your Step Goals. If your weekly average is around 9,000-13,000 steps/day or higher, you must be doing something intentional on a daily basis—values like these don't accumulate just from running to the bathroom several times a day, or from playing sports once a week! Personally, I can tell you that I accumulate many, many more steps on days that I exercise compared to days that I don't. Exercise is one of my personal strategies for meeting my Step Goal. That may not be your choice. The idea is to do what's right for you. Remember, the key to success with Manpo-kei is consistency—that is, accumulating a high number of steps on most, if not all days of the week, regardless of what you do to accumulate them.

Once you are able to sustain 9,000-13,000 steps/day week after week and you are ready for further improvements, I recommend bumping up the intensity and/or trying new activities for variety. Walk a little faster sometimes—consider jogging—play sports that require a little more exertion, etc. One of the advanced strategies I recommend is called Spike Days. Two or three days of the week work towards an elevated Step Goal. You choose what that unique Step Goal will be, but some people shoot for approximately 3,000-5,000 steps more than their usual Step Goal. Challenge yourself, but keep it comfortable so you are likely to do it again.

I also recommend some form of resistance training (e.g., weight lifting) in addition to pedometer self-monitoring. The number of steps/day you take are related to energy expenditure and general cardiovascular fitness—but resistance training provides the independent benefits of strength and shape—so the combined approach is best for maximizing health benefits. It is not the intent of this book to instruct you on the finer points of resistance training—once again, there are plenty of books out there! According to the experts, however, you should do some form of resistance training 2-3 times per week.

Manpo-kei rewards you with Bonus Steps for participation in resistance training and at least two other great types of exercise that pedometers cannot pick up, notably bicycling and swimming. Remember way back in the section on goal-setting I had you determine the number of steps you take in 10 minutes of continuous walking (see page 50). For convenience sake, let's say it was 1,000 steps. For every 10 minutes of continuous bicycling or swimming at a moderate intensity (similar to your continuous walk) add 1,000 steps to your day-end total. The same goes for resistance training. And for every 10 minutes you engage in vigorous bicycling or swimming, give yourself more Bonus Steps, equivalent to the number of steps you would take in 10 minutes of running. Just remember that it has to be 10 minutes of active time, not hanging out at the water fountain in the weight room, or clinging to the edge of the pool.

One more note. If you wear your pedometer to an aerobics class you may be dismayed when you notice how relatively few steps you get. Lifting your knee to your chin and waving your arms around above your head while simultaneously twisting your body and rising up on to your toes, will probably register as a step. All that for one measly step? Afraid so. Once again, I offer a Bonus Step plan to reflect the intensity of this activity. This plan is a little more complicated than the last. First, take off the pedometer (yes, I said off—so you don't double-count steps) and lock it safely in your locker while you're in class (I suspect pedometers will be easily led astray if separated from their masters). Go to class with your watch on and time the distinct sections of class (e.g., warm-up section, vigorous exercise, cool-down section). Then translate the times into Bonus Steps. For the warm-up section of class, give yourself the same number of steps as you would for the same time walking. During the vigorous dancing, stepping, jumping, hopping, shimmying, etc., give yourself the same number of steps as you would for the same time running. And finally, during the cool-down and any strengthening work, again give yourself the same number of steps you would for the same time walking. If you do this once or twice to get the feel for how long you spend doing what in your favorite classes, you'll come up with a number (say 8,000 steps in your hour-long funky dance class taught by that wild instructor Maria) that you credit to your day-end steps taken.

In the end, Manpo-kei is all about choice. The pedometer and Tracking Calendar lay it all out in front of you. These tools make it easy to manage your choices. You choose your Step Goals and the strategies you use to achieve them. You choose your Lowest Acceptable Level, how to deal with high-risk situations and counter relapse. You choose if you want to add Spike Days and give yourself Bonus Steps. You choose to do More Than Before. And you choose to wear the pedometer.

Remember Susan? She chose to wear a pedometer and practice Manpo-kei. Let's check in on her once again.

● ● ● ● ● ● ● ● ● ● ● ● ● ● ● ● ● ● ● ●

Cocktail Party Talk

As overheard at a holiday cocktail party—

Susan: Judith! You look fantastic! Tell me your secrets!

Judith: Well, I was so inspired by your success that I decided to push my Step Goal up for a couple of months.

Susan: Ah, yes, another practitioner of Manpo-kei! Do you have a pedometer on? I can't even see it! What were you shooting for?

Judith (smiling and patting her waist): 15,000. A complete Manko-pei Makeover. I walk to work part of the way everyday in addition to walking for exercise. I give myself Bonus Steps for swimming of course and I schedule at least one Spike Day a week. But you know, I love it. And I'm addicted now. I'm determined to get my Step Goal six days a week! On Sundays, though, I can't seem to manage more than around 5,000! Can you believe it—5,000!

Susan: Believe it, I lived it day after day! I was such a slug then. It seemed I was always busy, just not active apparently. I did the 15-20,000 thing when I was focused on losing weight. I had three Spike Days each week. But it isn't realistic for me for the long term. I maintain at about 8,500-9,500. And those are all intentional steps—I hardly get any incidental steps during my day. I do give myself Bonus Steps for weight training twice a week now, though. And my Lowest Acceptable Level is 6,500 steps. But I never seem to relapse anymore—I haven't been lower than 6,500 for four months now. I find it's easy to do More Than Before!

Judith: Well, I'm only planning the 15,000 thing for a couple more weeks—just 'til we get through the holidays. Then I'll probably drop down to 10-11,000 for maintenance. I have a sweet tooth—I need to keep my steps a bit on the high side at least five days a week. Times have changed though—seems we always used to try to exercise more after the holidays! But listen, the kids love their pedometers—they've actually given them names! And you know all the kids are wearing those homemade beaded idiot-strings now.

Susan: I know. It's funny isn't it. My husband calls his pedometer 'Peddy' and refers to it as 'he!' Poor guy, he's been doing a lot of office-work these last couple of weeks and can only make his Lowest Acceptable Level. He's due for a Booster Shot. He makes good choices though. He told me he would avoid the desserts tonight because his steps were so low today.

Judith (surveying the buffet table): Can you imagine how we used to make it through the holidays without Manpo-kei?

Susan: I shudder to think. Talk about a high-risk situation! All this food—I made sure to get 12,000 steps in before coming tonight. I likely won't be getting any more today! And I just love to sample a few of these indulgences!

Judith: Speaking of your husband, I just noticed him tapping 'Peddy' and motioning to you—I think he wants to hit the dance floor for a few extra steps! See ya later. By the way, you look great too! Continued luck with your Step Goals!

Susan: You know better than that—it's not about luck, Manpo-kei is about choice—and I choose to be naturally physically active!

Practitioner's Glossary

Baseline Activity Calendar - a 7-day calendar to be used during the first week of pedometer use, before behavior change is initiated.

Baseline Level - usual steps/day level before behavior change.

Bonus Steps - extra 'steps' added to day-end totals to account for activities that the pedometer is not sensitive to (e.g., bicycling, swimming, weight training).

Booster Shot - a process of re-assessment and re-commitment to Step Goals.

Current Steps/day - average steps/day changing weekly; reflects most recent accomplishment.

Decision-balance - a process of mentally preparing for behavior change by carefully weighing the pros and cons of the change.

Exercise - intentional structured physical activity done to improve physical fitness.

Goal-setting - a process of identifying a desired state or behavior (e.g., Step Goal) that you can work towards.

High-risk situation - one you recognize as potentially leading to a backslide in behavior.

Idiot-string - a string tied to a pedometer and attached to clothing with a safety pin (to keep from losing the pedometer).

Incidental activities - activities done for some purpose other than the activity itself.

Intentional activities - activities done primarily for the purpose of being active.

Lowest Acceptable Level (or Inactivity Index) - a number of steps/day that represents the minimum number of steps you will allow yourself.

Manpo-kei - a Japanese word originally referring to a pedometer as a '10,000 step meter', the term now refers to an individualized approach to increasing physical activity through a pedometer-based program of goal-setting and self-monitoring.

Manpo-kei Makeover - a change in lifestyle to increase steps/day.

More Than Before - a desired state when Current Steps/Day is greater than Baseline Level.

Naturally Active - a high level of lifestyle activity that may or may not include intentional exercise. It includes energy expended throughout the day in incidental work activities, chores, childcare, errands, commuting, etc.

Pedometer - a gadget that counts steps taken due to ambulatory activity.

Pedometer Accuracy Test - a quick test of pedometer performance that involves walking 20 steps and checking the pedometer for accurate recording.

Physical activity - any body movement, for whatever purpose.

Physical inactivity - a state in which bodily movement is minimal.

Refinement - a process of adjusting Step Goals and strategies.

Reflection - a process of carefully considering and explaining past behavior (e.g., day-end steps).

Relapse - three or more days of the week below your Lowest Acceptable Level.

Sedentarism - a lifestyle marked by much physical inactivity and relatively little physical activity.

SMART goals - a universal approach for assessing appropriateness of goals: Specific, Measurable, Attainable, Realistic, and Time-limited (or have an identifiable Time-frame).

Spike Days - an advanced Manpo-kei technique of setting an elevated Step Goal (above the usual Step Goal) a self-determined number of days/week.

Step Goal - a number of steps you want to attain by the end of the day.

Step Increment - any number of steps you add to your Baseline Level or Current Steps/day to obtain a new Step Goal

Strategies - the behaviors you practice to meet your Step Goal.

Tracking - a process of self-monitoring. In Manpo-kei, tracking is done using a combination of pedometers and calendars.

Tracking Calendar - a calendar to regularly track day-end steps and achievement of Step Goals. Can be used over the long-term or just for Booster Shots.

References

1. Flegal KM, Carrol MD, Kuczmarski RJ, Johnson CL. Overweight and obesity in the United States: Prevalence and trends, 1960-1994. Int J Obes Relat Metab Disord 1998;22(1):39-47.

2. Grundy SM, Blackburn G, Higgins M, Lauer R, Perri MG, Ryan D. Physical activity in the prevention and treatment of obesity and comorbidities. Med Sci Sports Exerc 1999;31(11 Suppl):S502-S508.

3. U.S. Department of Health and Human Services. Physical Activity and Health: A Report of the Surgeon General. Atlanta, GA: US Department of Health and Human Services, Centers for Disease Control and Prevention, National Center for Chronic Disease Prevention and Promotion; 1996.

4. Heini AF, Weinsier RL. Divergent trends in obesity and fat intake patterns: the American Paradox. Am J Med 1997;102(3):259-264.

5. Dietz WH. The role of lifestyle in health: the epidemiology and consequences of inactivity. Proc Nutri Soc 1996;55(3):829-840.

6. Ainsworth BE, Haskell WL, Whitt MC, Irwin ML, Swartz AM, Strath SJ, et al. Compendium of physical activities: An update of activity codes and MET intensities. Med Sci Sports Exerc 2000;32(Suppl 9):S498-S504.

7. U.S. Department of Health and Human Services. Healthy people 2000: Midcourse review and 1995 revisions. Washington, DC: Department of Health and Human Services; 1995.

8. Farrell SW, Kampert JB, Kohl HW, Barlow CE, Macera CA, Paffenbarger RS, et al. Influences of cardiorespiratory fitness levels and other predictors of cardiovascular disease in men. Med Sci Sports Exerc 1998;30(6):899-905.

9. Blair SN, Kampert JB, Kohl HW, Barlow CE, Macera CA, Paffenbarger RS, et al. Influences of cardiorespiratory fitness and other precursors on cardiovascular disease and all-cause mortality in men and women. JAMA 1996;276(3):205-210.

10. Dishman RK, Sallis SF. Determinants and interventions for physical activity and exercise. In: Bouchard C, Shephard R, Stephens T, editors. Physical activity, fitness and health: International proceedings and consensus statement. Champaign, IL: Human Kinetics; 1994.

11. Pate RR, Pratt M, Blair SN, Haskell WL, Macera CA, Bouchard C, et al. Physical activity and public health: a rec-ommendation from the Centers for Disease Control and

Prevention and the American College of Sports Medicine. JAMA 1995;273(5):402-407.

12. Gibbs-Smith C. The inventions of Leonardo da Vinci. London: Phaidon Press; 1978.

13. Hendelman D, Miller K, Baggett C, Debold E, Freedson P. Validity of accelerometry for the assessment of moderate intensity physical activity in the field. Med Sci Sports Exerc 2000;32(9):S442-S450.

14. Tudor-Locke CE, Myers AM. Methodological considerations for researchers and practitioners using pedometers to measure physical (ambulatory) activity. Res Q Exerc Sport 2001;72(1):1-12.

15. Tudor-Locke CE, Myers AM. Challenges and opportunities for measuring physical activity in sedentary adults. Sports Med 2001;31(312):91-100.

16. Hatano Y. Use of the pedometer for promoting daily walking exercise. ICHPER 1993;29:4-8.

17. Yamanouchi K, Takashi T, Chikada K, Nishikawa T, Ito K, Shimizu S, et al. Daily walking combined with diet therapy is a useful means for obese NIDDM patients not only to reduce body weight but also to improve insulin sensitivity. Diabetes Care 1995;18(6):775-778.

18. Tudor-Locke C, Ainsworth BE, Whitt MC, Thompson R, Addy CL, Jones DA. The relationship between pedometer-determined ambulatory activity and body composition variables. Int J Obes Relat Metab Disord 2001:25,1571-1578.

19. Rowlands AV, Eston RG, Ingledew DK. Relationship between activity levels, aerobic fitness, and body fat in 8- to 10-yr-old children. J App Physiol 1999;86(4):1428-1435.

20. McClung CD, Zahiri CA, Higa JK, Amstutz HC, Schmalzried TP. Relationship between Body Mass Index and activity in hip or knee arthroplasty patients. J Ortho Res 2000;18(1):35-39.

21. Tryon WW, Goldberg JL, Morrison DF. Activity decreases as percentage of overweight increases. Int J Obes Relat Metab Disord 1992;16(8):591-595.

22. Tudor-Locke C, Bell RC, Myers AM, Harris SB, Mitek N, Rodger NW. Pedometer-determined ambulatory activity in individuals with type 2 diabetes. Diabetes Res Clin Pract 2002; 55: 191-199.

23. Leermakers EA, Dunn AL, Blair SN. Exercise management of obesity. Med Clin North Am 2000;84(2):419-440.

24. Iwane M, Arita M, Tomimoto S, Satani O, Matsumoto M, Miyashita K, et al. Walking 10,000 steps/day or more reduces blood pressure and sympathetic nerve activity in mild essential hypertension. Hypertens Res 2000;23:573-580.

25. Sequeira MM, Rickenbach M, Wietlisbach V, Tullen B, Schutz Y. Physical activity assessment using a pedometer and its comparison with a questionnaire in a large population survey. Am J Epidemiol 1995;142(9):989-999.

26. Tudor-Locke C, Ainsworth BE, Popkin BM. Active commuting to school: An overlooked source of children's physical activity? Sports Med 2001;31(5):309-313.

27. Marcus BH, King TK, Clark MM, Pinto BM, Bock BC. Theories and techniques for promoting physical activity behaviours. Sports Med 1996;22(5):321-331.

28. Tudor-Locke CE, Myers AM, Rodger NW. Development of a theory-based daily activity intervention for individuals with Type 2 diabetes. Diabetes Educ 2001;27(1):85-93.

29. Tudor-Locke C, Jones GR, Myers AM, Paterson DH, Ecclestone NA. Contribution of structured exercise class participation and informal walking for exercise to daily physical activity in community-dwelling older adults. Res Q Exerc Sport in press.

Appendix A

Manpo-kei Shopping Checklist

◯ Small and lightweight

◯ Extended battery life

◯ Digital step-counter display
  *(neither distance nor calories are required for practitioners of
  Manpo-kei)*

◯ Secure attachment-clip
  The fewer buttons the better (remember, all you need is a step-counter)

◯ Protective cover
  (keeps reset button from being accidentally reset!)

◯ Cheap
  (expect $20-$60)

◯ Accurate
  (according to the in-store Pedometer Accuracy Test—see page 38)

Manpo-kei Baseline Activity Calendar

Monday	Tuesday	Wednesday	Thursday	Friday	Saturday	Sunday
Total Steps	Total Steps	Total Steps	Total Steps	Total Steps	Total Steps	Total Steps
Work Y N	Work Y N	Work Y N	Work Y N	Work Y N	Work Y N	Work Y N
Sport Y N	Sport Y N	Sport Y N	Sport Y N	Sport Y N	Sport Y N	Sport Y N
Exercise Y N	Exercise Y N	Exercise Y N	Exercise Y N	Exercise Y N	Exercise Y N	Exercise Y N
Type & Time	Type & Time	Type & Time	Type & Time	Type & Time	Type & Time	Type & Time

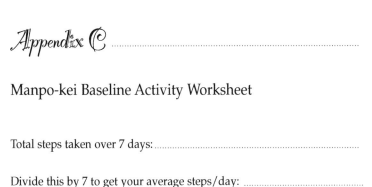

Manpo-kei Baseline Activity Worksheet

Total steps taken over 7 days:..

Divide this by 7 to get your average steps/day: ....

This is your Baseline Level.

Total steps accumulated over workdays and divide by the number of days you worked:..

Total steps accumulated over the weekend days and divide by 2:..............

Total up steps on the days you exercised and divide by the number of days you exercised: ....

Total up the steps on the days you did not exercise and divide by the number of days you did not exercise: ....

Manpo-kei Tracking Calendar

Step Goal	Monday	Tuesday	Wednesday	Thursday	Friday	Saturday	Sunday
	Steps Goal Y N	Steps Goal Y N	Steps Goal Y N	Steps Goal Y N	Steps Goal Y N	Steps Goal Y N	Steps Goal Y N
Step Goal	Monday	Tuesday	Wednesday	Thursday	Friday	Saturday	Sunday
	Steps Goal Y N	Steps Goal Y N	Steps Goal Y N	Steps Goal Y N	Steps Goal Y N	Steps Goal Y N	Steps Goal Y N
Step Goal	Monday	Tuesday	Wednesday	Thursday	Friday	Saturday	Sunday
	Steps Goal Y N	Steps Goal Y N	Steps Goal Y N	Steps Goal Y N	Steps Goal Y N	Steps Goal Y N	Steps Goal Y N
Step Goal	Monday	Tuesday	Wednesday	Thursday	Friday	Saturday	Sunday
	Steps Goal Y N	Steps Goal Y N	Steps Goal Y N	Steps Goal Y N	Steps Goal Y N	Steps Goal Y N	Steps Goal Y N

ISBN 155395481-5

9 781553 954811

1322988

Made in the USA